Essiac Herbal Tea Testimonials & Info

People tell how Essiac Tea helped them conquer their illness

by

Barry Bryant

1. I will start this book with my personal testimony.

In 1992 my friend Joe from Tampa was in critical condition with Lupus. He was on his death bed. I gave him some bottles of Essiac Tea. Within 2 months he was like a new man, totally energized and back to work. This made quite an impression on me.

In 2000 I had an enlarged prostate, and some nights I peed 15 times during the night. I was so exhausted from lack of sleep that I was always tired. Then I was diagnosed with prostate cancer. When I told my doctor that I was going to take Essiac Tea he got so angry at me that I thought that he was going to hit me! Well, I took my tea and my cancer went away. Now I pee once a night.

On June of 2019 my wife Denise was diagnosed with Stage 4 breast cancer. She really panicked. But she had confidence in my holistic knowledge. So she tried Essiac Tea. By December her doctor said that she was cancer-free. We monitor her condition carefully, and she continues to take the tea as a preventative.

Well, with this experience under my belt, I have decided to write a book of Essiac Tea testimonials. I will also briefly tell the story of how Essiac Tea came to be, as this is valuable knowledge.

First, the story of Essiac Tea:

2. The Story

Rene Caisse was a Canadian nurse who for a period of sixty years treated thousands of cancer patients with a herbal remedy.

In 1923 she discovered that one of her cancer patients, who had been officially declared incurable, made a complete recovery. This patient had taken an Ojibway herbal drink. Experimenting with other incurable cancer patients, Rene found that many of them recovered after starting a regimen of taking this Indian herbal drink twice daily.

Rene Caisse got the herbal formula from the Ojibway Indians. She named it Essiac. She then offered Essiac to terminal cancer patients. She documented thousands of cases of her patients who were cured of cancer. In 1937 the Royal Cancer Commission of Canada conducted hearings concerning Essiac. Rene Caisse's documented evidence was presented to the commission. The commission's conclusion was that Essiac was a cure for cancer.

The Canadian newspapers created such a furor about this one nurse's efforts that in 1938 the Canadian Parliament voted to let Rene use Essiac as a cure for cancer. The vote was close, but Essiac failed by three votes to be approved as an officially sanctioned cure for cancer.

In the 1960's Rene Caisse worked with the well-known Brusch Medical Clinic in Massachusetts. Dr. Brusch was the personal physician for President John F. Kennedy. After researching Essiac for 10 years, Dr. Brusch made the following statement: "Essiac is a cure for cancer, period. All studies done at laboratories in the United States and Canada support this conclusion." Further studies showed Essiac assisted other illnesses, such as AIDS, lupus, and multiple sclerosis.

It was, and always will be, one of my main goals to educate the public about Essiac. That is why I provide the formula for Essiac. I want you to know how to make it yourself. When enough of us know how to prepare and use Essiac, this knowledge can never be suppressed.

I researched every available bit of information about Essiac and Rene Caisse. We obtained our Essiac formula from Dr. Glum. The formula is presented to you in this book. This is the Essiac formula which was presented by Rene Caisse to the Royal Cancer Commission in 1937, and was later declared by the Royal Cancer Commission to "be a cure for cancer."

Sheila Snow, a Canadian researcher, has done a great job of preserving the truth about Essiac. She notes in her work that the Sheep Sorrel and the Burdock Root are the two "cancer killers" in the Essiac formula. They are the basic curative agents, and are the main ingredients. The other ingredients, Slippery Elm Bark and Rhubarb Root, "assist" the Sheep Sorrel and Burdock Root by increasing bile flow and assisting the intestinal tract to eliminate the toxins released by the Essiac. Simply put, the Sheep Sorrel and the Burdock Root do the curing, and the Slippery Elm and Rhubarb Root assist them to cure. Now we have also added small amounts of Kelp, Blessed Thistle, Red Clover and Watercress which Rene is reported to have used to "enhance" the curative power of her tea.

Over the years there has been great feedback as to the effectiveness of Essiac tea. Many people with Chronic Fatigue Syndrome, Lupus, Aids, Alzheimer's, and Multiple Sclerosis have successfully taken Essiac. Almost miraculous recoveries from Lupus and Chronic Fatigue have been reported to us. Multiple Sclerosis sufferers have reported less spectacular, but steady improvements in their conditions.

We live in an age of depleted immune systems. Overuse of antibiotics, overloading our bodies with toxins, pesticides, and chemicals, and years of improper nutrition have caused our immune systems to be exhausted and worn out. As Rene Caisse's herbal remedy rebuilds the body's immune system, the body is able to better overcome illness and fatigue.

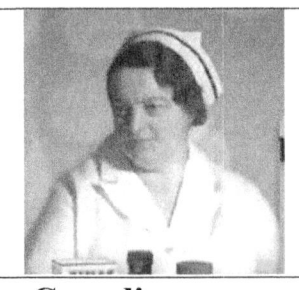

Canadian nurse Rene Caisse	Dr. Gary Glum

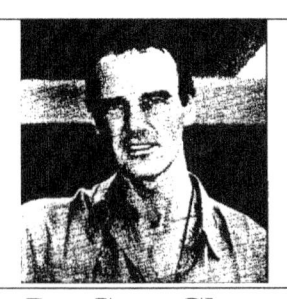

3. Why haven't you heard more about Essiac Tea?

You are not told the truth about the effectiveness of some cancer cures because of the business implications. You see, cancer is big business. And the big businesses that control the health care market protect their profits and interests. What many of us (myself included) have great difficulty accepting is that perhaps the medical establishment has placed a higher priority on profit making than they have curing cancer. This is hard to believe. It was for me. It is for others. I have many times spoken with cancer suffers who could not fathom that the institutions which they had trusted all of their lives would let them die in order to make more money. I appreciate their dilemma.

Many people, forced by the ravages of their steadily worsening cancer to choose whether or not to follow an alternative approach, elect not to. They seemingly would rather do this than accept that they have been betrayed. These people, rightly or wrongly, choose to stick by their cherished beliefs in their establishment, and thus do not venture out into the (for them) uncharted waters of alternative medicine. That is their choice, and I respect them for that. However I believe very strongly that it was important for them to have this choice. And that is the purpose of this book: to present this information to you so that you may have a choice. This is a fundamental right which is guaranteed to us by our beloved Constitution.

Some uncomfortable information is as follows: The largest industry in this country is the petrochemical industry. The second largest industry is cancer. Cancer is a $3.4 billion industry in this country. When a simple and inexpensive remedy for cancer exists, it threatens the livelihood of some very powerful institutions and groups of people. What about the FDA (Food and Drug Administration)? The FDA is controlled and funded by politicians. Politicians are controlled and funded by powerful institutions such as the drug companies and the AMA. The AMA has the largest lobbying group in Washington. The FDA periodically swoops down to eradicate approaches to curing cancer which are not approved by the FDA. However when cures for cancer which contain herbs or other natural ingredients are presented to the FDA for review, the FDA refuses to consider them because it only approves drugs. This "Catch 22" means that you will never see an alternative approach to curing cancer approved by them. In addition, they have set up a bureaucratic maze such that hundreds of millions of dollars are needed to fund the many studies which are required for FDA approval. Only the large drug companies can play this game.

What about your doctor? Your doctor places his career in jeopardy if he ever recommends a non-drug approach (non-FDA approved) to curing your cancer. At the turn of the century, the same monied interests which owned the major drug companies established the American Medical Association (AMA). While we were being told that the AMA was our protector against quackery, the AMA quietly but effectively launched a campaign to eradicate all approaches to medicine which competed with the use of drugs (allotropic medicine). Thus naturopathy, herbal medicine, and many other modalities faded from view. Meanwhile the AMA also quietly but steadily influenced the curriculums of the medical schools so that most doctors today are for the most part only taught a drug approach to healing. As an example, one doctor told me that, during his eight years of medical study, he received only four hours of nutrition training. So it isn't that your doctor is a bad guy. On the contrary, he or she is probably very hard working and dedicated. It is just that the system is just as aligned against him as it is against you when it comes to alternative approaches to medicine.

Some doctors are fighting this system. My hero is Dr. David G. Williams of PO Box 929, Ingram, Texas 78025. He publishes a fantastic newsletter called Alternatives for the Health Conscious Individual. I highly recommend this newsletter. Dr. Williams explains the medical establishment's control very succinctly: he says that if there is an effective cure that is inexpensive, and cannot be controlled by the AMA or the drug companies, you are not going to hear about it from your family doctor or the government.

4. Essiac Testimonials

I have gathered together testimonials from various sources. Therefore the formats vary widely. Please be patient here, but these are genuine personal reports from many various people.

a. Taken from *Well Being Journal* Vol. 7, No.2, March/April/98

THERE CAME A QUICK RAPPING at my door. It was the postman delivering a certified letter. With my hand shaking and my heart beating a mile a minute, I reached for the letter. My eyes riveted on the return address for a clue as to where it came from, I recognized the name of the surgeon's office where I had recently gone to get my breasts examined. At the time of the examination, the doctor had suggested that I set a date for surgery before leaving the office. I had done that. But, having second thoughts, I had phoned and canceled the appointment.

I ripped open the letter and read: "I am certain that you understood when I explained my concern to you. The radiologist in my office stated that there is a large mass in the left breast which is different from the other tissue. It is recommended that the mass be excised." The letter went on to say that I needed to phone and reschedule an appointment for surgery. It was signed by the doctor. I was petrified, but for some inexplicable reason I was in no hurry to have surgery.

For several months, I had been feeling a fullness in my right breast, and both breasts were sore to the touch. When I had gone for my regular mammogram, the technician told me I wouldn't be getting the results until the end of the week, in spite of the fact that the radiologist read the x-rays in the morning. I knew I was going to be on edge every time the phone rang.

I went for my annual gynecological checkup. The doctor said my right breast should be checked by a surgeon. It felt denser than it had the previous year. I was given the names of several surgeons whom I might call.

My husband drove me about fifty miles from our home to see a doctor I had chosen from the list. The doctor and an assistant examined me. The examination was painful due to the pressure they put on my breasts. They were trying to see if any fluid would come out. It didn't.

My complaint had actually begun with the right breast, but the in-house radiologist studied the mammograms I had brought with me and decided that it was actually the left breast that was showing a change. The doctor described what I had as a large mass, and he recommended that I have a lumpectomy per-formed on my left breast. I was smiling and joking while the doctor explained it to me. The doctor, however, did not smile. That led me to conclude this was serious business.

At first, I felt happy about the idea of getting rid of a big lump. Then the doctor mentioned that scar tissue would probably form where the lump was excised, and that the removal would not prevent another lump from growing in the same place. I thought to myself, "Surgery seems to be a no-win situation."

I was told I needed to cut out caffeine, take vitamin E, and start taking oil of primrose on a daily basis. I could buy what I needed at a health food store. It was also suggested I discontinue hormone replacement therapy.

I was alarmed when the doctor suggested that I might have to be placed on a male hormone to get rid of the pain. The last thing I wanted for myself was to look masculine. I pictured hair growing on my face. I thought to myself that I would rather be dead than turn into a freak.

The next day, my husband drove me to a nearby health food store to buy the vitamin E and other items I needed. We ran into a women who had helped him with some health problems he had once had. She told us about Essiac tea. She said many people had come into the store asking for it, and that they had had wonderful results. She was so enthusiastic about it that I thought to myself, "I can try it, and go under the knife later, if I decide to.

Early the next morning, I started on the program of drinking Essiac tea. It was to be consumed on an empty stomach once in the morning and again before I went to sleep. The tea had been used in Canada to cure cancer. I didn't know for sure that I had cancer, but the doctor had described what I had as a large mass.

Essiac tea had been used by a Canadian nurse, Rene Caisse, to successfully treat thousands of cancer patients from 1920 until her death in 1978. The treatment brought remissions to hundreds of documented cases, and the tea came within three' votes of being legalized by the Canadian parliament in 1938. The tea had the support of many prominent physicians, including a well-known doctor in the United States by the name of Dr. Charles Brusch. He is known for the prestigious Brusch Medical Center and for treating President Kennedy. He claimed a personal cure for cancer in his lower abdomen using the tea.

The main ingredients of Essiac tea are burdock root, turkey rhubarb root, sheep sorrel, and slippery elm bark. In 1966, two Hungarian scientists reported "considerable anti-tumor activity with the burdock root. In 1984, Japanese scientists discovered the mixture to be capable of reducing cell mutation. The Japanese named the new property they found in burdock root "the B-factor," for burdock factor. Essiac tea breaks down nodular masses to more normal tissue, while greatly alleviating pain.

Rene Caisse found that the tea reduced tumor growth and that the other herbs acted as blood purifiers, carrying destroyed tissue as well as infections thrown off by the malignancy out of the body. It was observed that the tea also strengthened the body's defense mechanisms, enabling normal cells to destroy abnormal ones as nature intended. If a tumor did not disappear, at least it could be regressed, then surgically removed after six to eight Essiac treatments. Yes, I believed I would take a chance on the tea, and go under the knife later, if I decide to.

The next morning, I awakened when it was still dark outside and I ingested the tea on an empty stomach. After breakfast, I took vitamin E, oil of primrose, and some multiple vitamins. During the day, I took vitamin C. There are orange groves near where we live, and my husband began making fresh orange juice every morning. At night, before I went to sleep, I ingested Essiac tea on an empty stomach. This regimen went on for six weeks.

During the treatment, a feeling of confidence came over me. I realized that 1 was no longer afraid about my breast. I put off calling the surgeon's office to reschedule the surgery. I had peace about doing this.

After taking the tea for six weeks, I noticed a remarkable improvement in my breasts. The pain I had experienced had disappeared one week after I had begun taking the tea. I also noticed the breast tissue seemed softer and mote supple. This was more the way breast tissue is supposed to feel. Before taking the tea, my breast had felt dense, lumpy, and hard. I hadn't been able to lay on my stomach because of the pain. After the treatment, I definitely noticed an improvement.

There was only one side effect with the tea: a constant itchy feeling on my arms and other parts of my body. I stopped taking the tea for two weeks, then took it again for six weeks. I again stopped for two weeks and then did another six weeks. I had peace about my breasts. I went on with my life and forgot about it until it was time once again for my annual mammogram.

The week after the mammogram, an envelope came in the mail. I opened the envelope and read: "We have reviewed the radiologist's report of your recent mammogram. There is no evidence of malignancy, and although this does not guarantee that there is no cancer, it is reassuring."

My heart leapt with joy, but I still wanted to make sure. I got on the phone and requested the radiologist's report. When it came, I read the words: "No definite dominant mass or speculated density is identified." This was evidence that my breast tissue had improved since my last mammogram. I had good reason to rejoice.

KATHRYN HAYN is trained as a teacher. She has a master's degree in education and a learning handicap teaching credential. She has written a book on the subject of ADD.

b. Short and sweet testimonials

Testimonials from Essiac Users

I began taking Essiac for severe arthritis and severe fatigue. The results are unbelievable! I am doing everyday normal things that I haven't been able to accomplish for 10 years; 10 years that have taken a great toll on my life. Since I have been taking Essiac I have felt the years float away, and I have regained the feeling of youth again. I am <u>very</u> happy with the results. My daughter Donna Geary of Alta Loma gave me my first bottle. The results are wonderful. The results were also immediate. Thank you for this wonderful drink.

Lucy Claudine Gibson

Lakewood California

My Brother-in law gave me a bottle of Essiac. I enjoyed the taste, soon realized a 20 year stomach problem was gone. It gives me an all-around better feeling. I am 60 years old, and I work 7 days a week.

My nephew in Wisconsin learned that he had cancer. Sent him the book "Canada's Cancer Cure" about Essiac. He was unable to take Chemo because of other health problems. He takes the tea faithfully, and one year later all is in remission.

Robert W. Heath

Fenwick, Michigan

My friend was diagnosed with Lung Cancer. I took it upon myself to give him a book on Essiac. He returned the next day to tell me that he was interested, and I set him up with a supply. They had planned on Chemotherapy but first wanted to monitor the growth rate which consisted of periodic x-rays. The first sets of x-rays showed such slow (almost negligible) growth that they waited for the second set to confirm the situation. After the second set of x-rays, the doctor told Bob that if he had had such success with chemotherapy, he (the doctor) would have been pleased to take the credit for such improvement.

We are both grateful to the people who keep an open mind and heart to give cancer patients hope for cure. I deeply believe Essiac has helped cure Bob, and I'm much more comfortable using it rather than making no effort to stay healthy systemically. If you'd like to share this letter with anyone, you have our blessing.

Greg Krepala

292 Martin Ct.

Aptos CA 95003

I took Essiac for prostate cancer. Under doctor's orders I was given chemotherapy. I also took Essiac, and as a result the PSA rating went down below zero (0). I took the combination for 16 months and when it held below zero I quit the chemotherapy. Since then the PSA readings went like this:

October: 0.15

April: 0.37

October 0.58

April 0.73

I have been continuing to take Essiac.

Paul E. Roche

East Haven, Connecticut

I had ovarian cancer which was diagnosed as widespread. They removed my ovaries and six inches of colon. I was advised afterwards that they could not remove all of the cancer cells and they recommended chemotherapy. I refused because of heart problems (I had two heart surgeries the previous years). I had found an article about Essiac and told the doctors I was going to try it. Well the results have been <u>remarkable</u>. I had lost over sixty-two pounds, and have now gained over sixteen back. Have been stronger and able to resume my work with ceramics. I do not believe that I would be alive now if it had not been for Essiac. I recommend it to everyone, and I am amazed at how cancer touches so many lives.

Doris Kearns

Porter, Texas

ps: My last exam by the oncologist showed results which were "perfect, perfect". I feel wonderful.

I had breast cancer. I started taking Essiac 3 weeks prior to my first chemotherapy session. Every side effect that was predicted I would have were so-o-o diminished that I hardly noticed them. My blood work, both chemistry and hemo were, I was told, <u>FANTASTIC</u> for a chemotherapy patient. I play duplicate bridge with as many as 140 people attending a local game. Everyone commented on my appearance and energy level and were amazed. Some started taking Essiac for general health reasons. How do I know that it was Essiac? I went to California after my 5th chemo. and stayed for three weeks. Since we were moving from place to place, I did not take Essiac. Upon returning home I received my 6th and final treatment. I was so very sick: nausea, diarrhea, heartburn so bad that I couldn't sleep, and I was so very tired. I start radiation *in a week, and you can bet that I will not be without my Essiac.*

June K. Outerson

Phoenix, Maryland

c. **Handwritten Reports**

Fax Cover Letter

to	Natural Heritage Enterprises	fax no.	(407)8269524
from	Pawel Heydel/Warsaw - Poland	fax no.	004822-8467862
total number of pages, including cover letter	1	date	31 May 98

If you do not receive all pages, call telephone no. 004822-6420687

Dear Sirs,

I have read a very interesting publication "THE ESSIAC HANDBOOK" published in the Internet. I am also one of the "completely cured cases" - after one year of taking ESSIAC my cancer - to the complete astonishment of my doctors - was gone. Since it is difficult to get it in Poland I am asking if it is possible to order it from You and have it sent to Warsaw. I would be interested in 6 boxes of the dried herbal mixture for the beginning. Please let me know what would be the complete cost of this operation and if it is possible to pay with Master Card.
Many thanks for quick reply in advance

With best regards

Pawel Heydel

TESTIMONIAL LETTER

Date: 1/16/98

My name is Doris Kearns. My address is 22232 E. Martin, Porter, TX. 77365. My telephone number is _____.

On June, 1997, I began taking Essiac for the following conditions (illness): Ovarian Cancer. The results of using the Essiac are:

On May 10, 1997 I had cancer surgery which had been diagnosed as widespread. They removed ovaries and six inches of colon. I was advised afterwards that they could not remove all cells and recommended chemotherapy. I refused because of heart problems. Had two heart surgeries with three stents implant the previous year. I had found an article about Essiac and told the doctors I was going to try it. Well the results have been remarkable. I had lost over sixty two pounds and have now gained over fifteen back. Have been stronger and able to resume my work with ceramics. I do not believe I would be alive now if it had not been for Essiac. I recommend it to everyone and am amazed at how cancer touches so many lives. God bless you all.

Signature: Doris Kearns

Please mail to: Ravelco, 4118 Montrose Ct., Orlando FL 32812. Your assistance in writing this letter will help others learn the truth about Essiac. Thank you very much! Many will benefit from your experience.

Feb. 4, '98. Waited until last exam by oncologist and the _____ "Perfect Pap ck." I feel wonderful.

Hello Good People,

It's me again in need of more "Essiac Handbooks". I don't know why but I'm coming into contact with people with cancer regularly. Maybe it's one of Gods subtle ways of getting your information out to the people. It has helped one friend of mine who went through colon cancer like me and whipped it with doctors conventional means (which had strong aftereffects). One year later they diagnosed him with lung cancer. I took it upon myself this time to give him your book on Essiac. He returned the next day very interested and I set him up with a supply. They had planned on chemotherapy but first wanted to monitor the growth rate which consisted of periodic x-rays. Even the first set of x-rays showed such slow (almost negligable) growth they waited for the second set to confirm the situation. After the second set of x-rays, the doctor told "Bob" that if he had had such success with chemo-therapy, he (the doctor) would have been pleased to take the credit for such improvement. Since then Bob has aquired the Kumbacha starter from you and we both plan to make it a daily habit too.

We are both grateful to people like you who

TESTIMONIAL LETTER

Date: June 4, 1998

My name is Lucy Claudine Gibson. My address is 4638 Briercrest Ave. Lakewood, Calf. 90713. My telephone number is ( ).

On May 2, 1998, I began taking Essiac for the following conditions (illness): Severe Arthritis and severe fatigue. The results of using the Essiac are:

Unbelievable! I am doing every day normal things to do — but I haven't been able to accomplish this for years — 10 years has taken a great toll on living. Since I have been taking "Essiac" I have felt the years float away — and I have regained the feeling of youth again. I am very happy with the results. My daughter Donna Geary of Alta Loma gave me a bottle this last Mothers day. The results are wonderful. The results are also immediate. Thank you for this wonderful drink.

Please send me one bottle as I am 76 yrs old and on social security — if I could — I would buy a case of it.

Thanks again,

Lucy Claudine Gibson
4638 Briercrest Avenue
Lakewood, Calf 90713

P.S. I need a Phamplet discribing all the herbs!

Signature: _____

Please mail to: Ravelco, 4118 Montrose Ct., Orlando FL 32812: Your assistance in writing this letter will help others learn the truth about Essiac. Thank you very much! Many will benefit from your experience.

TESTIMONIAL LETTER

Date: _____

My name is Paul F. Roche, My address is 16 Glenwood Drive East Haven, CT 06512. My telephone number is (___) _____.

On Nov., 1993, _____ began taking Essiac for the following conditions (illness): Prostate Cancer. The results of using the Essiac are:

In August 1994, under doctor's orders I was given chemotherapy. I never told the doctor that I was taking Essiac and as a result the PSA rating went down below 0 (zero). I took the combination for 15 months and when it held below 0 I quit the chemotherapy. Since then the PSA reading go as this Oct 6, 1995 — 0.15

Apr. 7, 1996 — 0.37
Oct 4, 1996 — 0.58
Apr 1, 1997 — 0.73

The local supply of Essiac was uncertain, and when I saw your ad in Spotlight I ordered my first supply on 11/27/96. Except for a period when I was afflicted with Sciatica and had to take strong pain killers, I have been taking Essiac again. I have ordered a supply and expect to receive it soon.

Signature: Paul F. Roche

Please mail to: Ravelco, 4118 Montrose Ct., Orlando FL 32812: Your assistance in writing this letter will help others learn the truth about Essiac. Thank you very much! Many will benefit from your experience.

d. **Additional Information:**

Knowledge of Essiac may change your life. It may give you the knowledge to make more informed decisions for yourself and your loved ones concerning cancer, AIDS, and other prevalent diseases, which threaten every American family. I am hoping that this booklet will also give many of you enough knowledge and interest in the four common herbs of Rene's herbal formula so that you will seek out herbalists who can teach you how to identify, collect and process your own Essiac!

You may also, as I do, find yourself taking Rene's herbal remedy daily as a Preventative and Detoxifier.

In summary, the information contained herein is offered to you in the spirit of love and brotherhood. We hope that you accept it as such, process the information, and pass it along in the spirit of love and brotherhood!

In today's society we live with a lot of fear. It is my hope that your knowledge of Rene's work may better assist you to live without fear concerning several of our most dangerous diseases.

Dedication

This handbook is dedicated to Dr. Gary L. Glum, whose courageous struggle let the knowledge of Essiac be known to us.

More Background

Rene Caisse was a nurse in Canada. In 1923 she observed that one of her doctor's patients, a woman with terminal cancer, made a complete recovery. Inquiring into the matter, Rene found that the woman had cured herself with an herbal remedy which was given to her by an Ojibway Indian herbalist. Rene visited the medicine man, and he gladly and freely presented her with his tribe's formula. He explained that the Ojibway used their herbal remedy for both spiritual balance and body healing. The formula consisted of four common herbs. They were blended and cooked in a fashion which caused the concoction to have greater curative power than any of the four herbs themselves. The four herbs were

Sheep Sorrel, Burdock Root, Slippery Elm Bark, and Rhubarb Root.

With her doctor's permission, Rene began to administer the herbal remedy to other terminal cancer patients who had been given up by the medical profession as incurable. Most recovered.

Rene then began to collect the herbs herself, prepare the remedy in her own kitchen, and to treat hundreds of cancer cases. She found that Essiac, as she named the herbal remedy, could not undo the effects of severe damage to the life support organs. In such cases, however, the pain of the illness was alleviated and the life of the patients was extended longer than predicted. In the other cases, where the life support organs had not been severely damaged, cure was complete, and the patients lived another 35 or 40 years.

Rene selflessly dedicated herself to helping these patients. She continued to treat hundreds of patients from her home. She did not charge for her services. Donations were her only income. They barely kept her above the poverty line. Over the years word of her work began to spread. The Canadian medical establishment did not take kindly to this nurse administering this remedy directly to anyone with cancer who requested her help. Thus began many years of harassment and persecution by the Canadian Ministry of Health and Welfare. Word of this struggle was carried throughout Canada by newspapers.

The newspaper coverage of Rene's work began to make her famous throughout Canada. Word was also spread by the families of those healed by Essiac. Eventually, the Royal Cancer Commission became interested in her work. They undertook to study Essiac.

In 1937 the Royal Cancer Commission conducted hearings about Essiac. Their conclusion was that Essiac was a cure for cancer.

Eventually the Canadian Parliament, prodded by the newspaper coverage and the widespread support generated for Rene by former patients and grateful families, voted in 1938 on legislation to legalize the use of Essiac. Fifty-five thousand signatures were collected on a petition presented to the Parliament. The vote was close, but Essiac failed by three votes to be approved as an officially sanctioned cure for cancer.

The complete story of Rene Caisse's life and struggles is told in a book written by Dr. Gary L. Glum entitled The Calling of An Angel. It tells of the documented recovery of thousands of cancer patients who had been certified in writing by their doctors as incurable. Rene continued her work for 40 years until her death in 1978. Rene had entrusted her formula to several friends, one of whom passed the formula along to Dr. Glum.

Of interest is that, in the 1960s, Rene Caisse worked with the well-known Brusch Clinic in Massachusetts. Dr. Charles A. Brusch was the personal physician for President John F. Kennedy. After 10 years of research about Essiac, Dr. Brusch made the following statement: "Essiac is a cure for cancer, period. All studies done at laboratories in the United States and Canada support this conclusion." A testimonial letter from Dr. Brusch is included in this handbook.

We are very indebted to Dr. Glum for his work.

What Essiac Is

Rene Caisse's original herbal formula contains four commonly occurring herbs:

Sheep Sorrel (Rumex acetosella).

Burdock Root (Arctium lappa).

Slippery Elm (Ulcus fulva).

Turkey Rhubarb (Rheum palmatum).

The Formula

Ingredients:

52 parts: Burdock Root (cut or dried) (parts by weight)

16 parts: Sheep Sorrel (powdered)

1 part: Turkey Rhubarb (powdered) or 2 parts domestic Rhubarb

4 parts: Slippery Elm (powdered)

This is the basic four herb formula which was presented to the Royal Cancer Commission in 1937 and was found by them to be "a cure for cancer". Later in her life, while working with Dr. Charles Brusch in Massachusetts, Rene added small potentizing amounts of four other herbs to her basic four herb formula. As provided to us by a woman who worked with Rene, and was given the formula by Rene, these extra four herbs were added as follows: Kelp (2 parts), Red Clover (1 part), Blessed Thistle (1 part), Watercress (0.4 parts). We consider the addition of these four extra herbs optional.

Supplies Needed:

4 gallon stainless steel pot with lid 3 gallon stainless steel pot with lid Stainless steel fine mesh double strainer, funnel & spatula 12 or more 16 oz. sterilized amber glass bottles with airtight caps, or suitable substitutes.

Preparation:

1. Mix dry ingredients thoroughly. Place herbs in a plastic bag and shake vigorously. Herbs are light sensitive; keep stored in a cool dark place.

2. Bring 2 gallons of sodium free distilled water to a rolling boil in the 4 gallon pot (with lid on). Should take approximately 30 minutes at sea level.

3. Stir in 1 cup of dry ingredients. Replace lid and continue to boil for 10 minutes.

4. Turn off stove. Scrape down the sides of the pot with the spatula and stir mixture thoroughly. Replace the lid.

5. Allow the pot to remain closed for 12 hours. Then turn the stove to the highest setting and heat to <u>almost</u> a boil (approximately 20 minutes). Do not let boil.

6. Turn off the stove. Strain the liquid into the 3 gallon pot. Clean the 4 gallon pot and strainer. Then strain the filtered liquid back into the 4 gallon pot.

7. Use the funnel to pour the hot liquid into sterilized bottles immediately, and tighten the caps. After the bottles have cooled, retighten the caps.

8. Refrigerate. Rene's herbal drink contains no preservative agents. If mold should develop, discard the bottle immediately.

Caution: All bottles and caps must be sterilized after use if you plan to reuse them for Essiac. Bottle caps must be washed and rinsed thoroughly, and may be cleaned with a 3% solution of <u>food grade</u> hydrogen peroxide (may be purchased in health food stores). To make a 3% solution, mix 1 ounce of 35% food grade hydrogen peroxide with 11 ounces of sodium free distilled water. Let soak for 5 minutes, rinse and dry. If food grade hydrogen peroxide is not available, use one half teaspoon of Clorox to one gallon of distilled water.

Instructions for Use (as reported by Dr. Glum)

1. Keep refrigerated.

2. Shake bottle well before using.

3. May be taken either cold from the bottle, or warmed (never microwave).

4. As a Preventative, daily take 4 tablespoons (2 ounces) at bedtime or on an empty stomach at least 2 hours after eating.

5. Cancer and AIDS sufferers, or other ill people, may wish to twice daily take 4 tablespoons (2 ounces), once in the morning, 5 minutes before eating, and once in the evening, at least 2 hours after eating.

Note:

>a. Stomach Cancer patients must dilute the herbal drink with an equal amount of sodium free distilled water.

b. Many people have reported that Rene's drink works well to detoxify the body, and have taken it as a detoxification program.

<u>Precaution</u>: Some doctors advise against taking the herbal formula while pregnant.

<u>Recommendation</u>: Rene reported that the twelve hour brewing process is essential for Essiac to have its special powers. Essiac is being offered to the public in pills, teabags, and homeopathic drops. We do not recommend them. They may work, but they are not what Rene Caisse used, nor have we seen evidence that they work.

What It Does

The components of Rene's herbal drink interact to have an amazing effect on the human body. The chemicals, minerals, and vitamins all act synergistically together to produce a variety of healing agents.

Sheep Sorrel:

Sorrel plants have been a folk remedy for cancer for centuries both in Europe and America. Sheep Sorrel has been observed by researchers to break down tumors, and to alleviate some chronic conditions and degenerative diseases.

It contains high amounts of vitamins A and B complex, C, D, E, K, P and vitamin U. It is also rich in minerals, including calcium, chlorine, iron, magnesium, silicon, sodium, sulfur, and has trace amounts of copper, iodine, manganese and zinc. The combination of these vitamins and minerals nourishes all of the glands of the body. Sheep Sorrel also contains carotenoids and chlorophyll, citric, malic, oxalic, tannic and tartaric acids.

The chlorophyll carries oxygen throughout the bloodstream. Cancer cells do not live in the presence of oxygen. It also:

- reduces the damage of radiation burns
- increases resistance to X-rays
- improves the vascular system, heart function intestines, and lungs
- aids in the removal of foreign deposits from the walls of the blood vessels
- purifies the liver, stimulates the growth of new tissue
- reduces inflammation of the pancreas, stimulates the growth of new tissue
- raises the oxygen level of the tissue cells

Sheep Sorrel is the primary healing herb in Essiac.

Burdock Root

For centuries Burdock has been used throughout the world to cure illness and disease. The root of the Burdock is a powerful blood purifier. It clears congestion in respiratory, lymphatic, urinary and circulatory systems. It promotes the flow of bile, and eliminates excess fluid in the body. It stimulates the elimination of toxic wastes, relieves liver malfunctions, and improves digestion. The Chinese use Burdock Root as an aphrodisiac, tonic, and rejuvenator. It assists in removing infection from the urinary tract, the liver, and the gall bladder. It expels toxins through the skin and urine. It is good against arthritis, rheumatism, and sciatica.

Burdock Root contains vitamins A, B complex, C, E, and P. It contains high amounts of chromium, cobalt, iron, magnesium, phosphorus, potassium, silicon, and zinc, and lesser amounts of calcium, copper, manganese, and selenium.

Much of the Burdock Roots curative power is attributed to its principal ingredient of Unulin, which helps to strengthen vital organs, especially the liver, pancreas, and spleen.

Slippery Elm Inner Bark

Slippery Elm Bark is widely known throughout the world as an herbal remedy. As a tonic it is known for its ability to sooth and strengthen the organs, tissues, and mucous membranes, especially the lungs and stomach. It promotes fast healing of cuts, burns, ulcers and wounds. It revitalizes the entire body.

It contains, as its primary ingredient, a mucilage, as well as quantities of garlic acid, phenols, starches, sugars, the vitamins A, B complex, C, K, and P. It contains large amounts of calcium, magnesium, and sodium, as well as lesser amounts of chromium and selenium, and trace amounts of iron, phosphorous, silicon and zinc.

Slippery Elm Bark is known among herbalists for its ability to cleanse, heal, and strengthen the body.

Rhubarb

Rhubarb, also a well-known herb, has been used worldwide since 220 BC as a medicine.

The Rhubarb root exerts a gentle laxative action by stimulating the secretion of bile into the intestines. It also stimulates the gall duct to expel toxic waste matter, thus purging the body of waste bile and food. As a result, the liver is cleansed, and chronic liver problems are relieved.

Rhubarb root contains vitamin A, many of the B complex, C, and P. Its high mineral content includes calcium, chlorine, copper, iodine, iron, magnesium, manganese, phosphorous, potassium, silicon, sodium, sulfur, and zinc.

Rene Caisse's Herbal Drink Has The Following Therapeutic Activity:

1. Prevents the buildup of excess fatty deposits in artery walls, heart, kidney and liver.

2. Regulates cholesterol levels by transforming sugar and fat into energy.

3. Destroys parasites in the digestive system and throughout the body.

4. Counteracts the effects of aluminum, lead and mercury poisoning.

5. Strengthens and tightens muscles, organs and tissues.

6. Makes bones, joints, ligaments, lungs, and membranes strong and flexible, less vulnerable to stress or stress injuries.

7. Nourishes and stimulates the brain and nervous system.

8. Promotes the absorption of fluids in the tissues.

9. Removes toxic accumulations in the fat, lymph, bone marrow, bladder, and alimentary canals.

10. Neutralizes acids, absorbs toxins in the bowel, and eliminates both.

11. Clears the respiratory channels by dissolving and expelling mucus.

12. Relieves the liver of its burden of detoxification by converting fatty toxins into water-soluble substances that can then be easily eliminated through the kidneys.

13. Assists the liver to produce lecithin, which forms part of the myelin sheath, a white fatty material that encloses nerve fibers.

14. Reduces, perhaps eliminates, heavy metal deposits in tissues (especially those

surrounding the joints) to reduce inflammation and stiffness.

15. Improves the functions of the pancreas and spleen by increasing the effectiveness of insulin.

16. Purifies the blood.

17. Increases red cell production, and keeps them from rupturing.

18. Increases the body's ability to utilize oxygen by raising the oxygen level in the tissue cells.

19. Maintains the balance between potassium and sodium within the body so that the fluid inside and outside each cell is regulated: in this way, cells are nourished with nutrients and are also cleansed.

20. Converts calcium and potassium oxalates into a harmless form by making them solvent in the urine. Regulates the amount of oxalic acid delivered to the kidneys, thus reducing the risk of stone formation in the gall bladder, kidneys, or urinary tract.

21. Protects against toxins entering the brain.

22. Protects the body against radiation and X-rays.

23. Relieves pain, increases the appetite, and provides more energy along with a sense of well being.

24. Speeds up wound healing by regenerating the damaged area.

25. Increases the production of antibodies like lymphocytes and T-cells in the thymus gland, which is the defender of our immune system.

26. Inhibits and possibly destroys benign growths and tumors.

27. Protects the cells against free radicals.

Essiac and Chronic Fatigue, Lupus, Alzheimer's, Etc.

We have found Essiac to be very helpful to many people with Chronic Fatigue Syndrome, Lupus, Multiple Sclerosis, and Alzheimer's. To the best of our knowledge, all Lupus suffers who have taken Essiac have been significantly helped. We have also witnessed very rapid recoveries among chronic fatigue sufferers. Usually they report a very dramatic increase in energy. Some multiple sclerosis sufferers had less dramatic, but steady improvements in their conditions. One lady put her crutches away after taking Essiac for three months. Alzheimer's sufferers have reported improvements. Some with arthritis have reported improvement, although apparently not all arthritic sufferers are helped by Essiac.

It appears that Essiac's actions to remove heavy metals, detoxify the body, restore energy levels, and rebuild the immune system, all act to restore the body to a level to where it is able to better defeat the illness. In other words, Essiac rebuilds the immune system and improves the illness defeating ability of the body so that it can then rid itself of the illness.

Essiac and AIDS

In 1993 Dr. Gary Glum worked with an AIDS project in Los Angeles. The project had sent 179 AIDS patients home to die. They had pneumocystis carinii and histoplasmosis. Their weight was down and their cell counts were less than ten.

The project gave Dr. Glum five of these patients to work with. He took them off AZT and put them on a protocol of taking 2 ounces of Essiac three times a day. By February of

1994, all of the other patients had died. Dr. Glum's five patients were still alive. They were exercising, eating three meals a day, their weights were back to normal, and they had no appearance of illness.

An Endorsement by Dr. Julian Whitaker, M.D.

Dr. Julian Whitaker publishes a very informative and enlightening monthly newsletter named Health & Healing. It has 430, OOO subscribers. In his November, 1995 issue he has an article titled "What I Would Do If I Had Cancer". He states that if he had cancer, he personally would follow a regimen which included changing his diet, taking the nutritional supplements Vitamin C, Shark Cartilage, Coenzyme Q1O, and he would take Essiac tea.

Dr. Whitaker has over twenty years of experience. He has written five major health books: *Reversing Heart Disease, Reversing Diabetes, Reversing Health Risks, A Guide to Natural Healing, and Is Heart Surgery Necessary?* Dr. Whitaker directs the Whitaker Wellness Institute in Newport Beach, California, which has treated thousands of patients. Should you desire information about subscribing to his newsletter, call (800)705-5559.

I highly recommend this newsletter to anyone who has a serious illness and wishes to become more knowledgeable about the complete range of healing modalities which are available. He also proscribes a 7 step 30 day wellness program "that will turn your life around".

Random Quotes from Rene Caisse:

"Though I worked each day from 9am to 9pm, my work was so absorbing there was no sense of fatigue. My waiting room was a place of happiness where people exchanged their experiences and shared their hope. After a few treatments, patients seemed to throw off their depression, fear, and distress. Their outlook became optimistic and as their pain decreased, they became happy and talkative."

"I could see the changes in some of the patients. A number of them, presented to me by their doctors after everything known to medical science had been tried and failed, being literally carried into my clinic for their first treatment. To later see these same people walk in on their own, after only five or six treatments, more than repaid me for all of my endeavors. I have helped thousands of such people. Some weeks I would have five or six hundred patients. I offered the treatment at no charge."

"Most importantly, and this was verified in animal tests conducted at the Brusch Medical Center and other laboratories, it was discovered that one of the most dramatic effects of taking this remedy was its affinity for drawing all of the cancer cells, which had spread, back to the original site at which point the tumor would first harden, then later soften until it vanished altogether. In other cases, the tumor would decrease in size to where it could be surgically removed with minimal complications. "

Bibliography & Reading List

The Calling of an Angel by Dr. Gary Glum, 1988, Silent Walker Publishing, PO Box 80098, Los Angeles CA, 90080 Tel: (310) 271 9931

The Essence of Essiac by Sheila Snow, 1993

Essiac: Nature's Cure For Cancer: An Interview with Dr. Gary Glum by Elisabeth Robinson, "Wildfire Magazine", Vol. 6, No. 1

Cancer Therapy by Ralph W. Moss, Ph.D., Equinox Press, 331 W. 57th St., Suite 268, New York, NY 10019, 1992

Health & Healing newsletter by Dr. Julian Whitaker, Phillips Publishing, 7811 Montrose Rd., Potomac MD 20854

My Favorite Source to Purchase Essiac Tea:

I purchase my Essiac tea from the following company in the United States. They give me courteous attention when I telephone them, their Essiac tea is made from organic herbs of the highest quality, their service is good, and their prices are fair.

Essiac can be purchased from:

Natural Heritage Enterprises
www.remedies.net   Tel: 719 256 4876

Their Products and Prices:

1. Bottles of Rene Caisse's Herbal Remedy: Bottles of the herbal remedy can be purchased by mail order for US$14.50 per 16 oz. bottle. Made using only organic herbs, with rigid adherence to Rene's formula (her basic 4 herb formula enhanced with the additional 4 potentizing herbs).

2. **Dried Herbal Mix:** Should you wish to prepare your own Rene Caisse herbal drink, you may mail order packets of the dried herb combination. Each packet will allow you to prepare approximately one half gallon of the drink. The cost is US$12.00 per packet.

Charles A. Brusch, M.D.
15 Grozier RD.
Cambridge, Massachusetts 02138

April 6, 1990

TO WHOM IT MAY CONCERN:

Many years have gone by since I first experienced the use of ESSIAC with my patients who were suffering from many varied forms of Cancer.

I personally monitored the use of this old therapy along with

Rene Caisse R.N. whose many successes were widely reported. Rene worked with me at my medical clinic in Cambridge, Massachusetts and where, under the supervision of my many medical doctors on staff, she proceeded with a series of treatments on terminal Cancer patients and laboratory mice and together we refined and perfected her formula.

On mice it has been shown to cause a decided recession of the mass and a definite change in cell formation.

Clinically, on patients suffering from pathologically proven Cancer, it reduces pain and causes a recession in the growth. Patients gained weight and showed a great improvement in their general health. Their elimination improved considerably and their appetite became whetted.

Remarkably beneficial results

were obtained even those cases at the "end of the road" where it proved to prolong life and the "quality" of that life.

In some cases, if the tumor didn't disappear, it could be surgically removed after ESSIAC with less risk of metastases resulting in new outbreaks.

Hemorrhage has been rapidly brought under control in many difficult cases, open lesions of lip and breast responded to treatment, and patients with Cancer of the stomach have returned to normal activity among many other remembered cases. Also, intestinal burns from radiation were healed and damage replaced, and it was found to greatly improve whatever the condition.

All these patient cases were diagnosed by reputable physicians and surgeons.

I do knew that I have witnessed

in my clinic and knew of many other cases where ESSIAC was the therapy used, a treatment which brings about restoration through destroying the tumor tissue and improving the mental outlook which reestablishes physiological function.

I endorse this therapy even today for I have in fact cured my own Cancer, the original site of which was the lower bowel, through ESSIAC alone.

My last Pete examination, where I Aces expedited throughout the intestinal tract while hospitalized (August, 1989) for a hernia problem, no sign of malignancy was found.

Medical documents validate this.

I have taken ESSIAC every day since my diagnosis (1984) and my recent examination has given me a clear bill of health.

I remained a partner with Rene repose until her death in 1978 and was the only person who had her complete trust and to whom she confided her knowledge and "know-howl of what she named 'ESSIAC."

Others have imitated, but a minor success rate should never be accented when the true therapy available.

Executed as a legal document.

Charles A. Brusch

Editor's Note: Dr. Brusch was President John F. Kennedy's personal physician

---

MORE ESSIAC TESTIMONIALS

In the fall of 1992 my mother who lives in Ohio was told that her throat and lung cancer had reached the point that she only had ninety days left to live. My sister and I began to help her straighten out her affairs. I heard about Mountain Magic Essiac. I sent her some. She drank it for two months. On December 22, she went back to visit the doctor. He thought that she was coming in to say goodbye. When he checked her, she was in total remission. I am a nurse, and I kept her x-rays as proof of her recovery.

Ellen Broderick
Winter Springs, Florida

I started taking your Essiac several months ago. The results have been Profound and Dramatic. Thank you.

John Tolleson
Columbus, Ohio

My uncle had lung cancer. They gave him six months to live. He started taking Essiac. That was four years ago. He is convinced that the Essiac saved him.

Rhonda M.M
Harrison, Ohio

My friend Joe Roberts was in a very bad way with Lupus. He could hardly move about. Some thought he was close to death. I gave him two bottles of Mountain Magic herbal tea (Essiac). He improved, and started taking Essiac. Within a month he looked like a new man, and appeared completely healed.

Martha Mylander
Gainsville, Florida

I had prostate cancer. My doctor gave me six months. I took Mountain Magic, as well as several other natural cures. My prostate cancer is gone.

A liquor store manager in Detroit, Michigan

My husband has been through every treatment for his illness, and I am now trying Essiac tea. I thought I would try it first for my various aches and pains, stress, etc. I believe it has done wonders for me so I have started giving him the tea. It won't hurt and maybe his life will be better. A friend of mine has liver cancer and even though the onco. gave him six months he is now going on two years and says the only thing he takes is Essiac tea. Believe me, he is living proof of its success for him.

Betty at MPIP Bulletin Board July 18, 1997

I met a member of the Natural Heritage company at a seminar. He told me about Essiac. I had a cancerous condition in my female organs which was causing me a lot of pain. I took the Essiac, my pain went away, and I am now free of cancer. God Bless Natural Heritage Enterprises! My eyes are now opened up to the value of natural healing systems, and I spend a lot of time preaching this new religion to my friends.

Marjorie L.
Stuart, Florida

I am 71 years old. I have had a very rare illness for twenty years. The medical people don't know what causes it, and they don't have a cure. It is called Cogan's Syndrome. It has destroyed my hearing in both ears, caused a lot of vertigo, a lot of aches and pain, and has damaged my heart. Most of my life I have had several colds every year and usually a case of the flu. In January of 1996, the flu turned into pneumonia. That was when I decided to give your Mountain Magic tea a try.

I am happy to tell you that since I began using your Mountain Magic I have not had a cold or a sign of the flu. I do believe that it has helped in my recovery from the pneumonia. I plan to continue its use. I drink 2 ounces about three times a week.

Calvin Goranson
299 Lake Mamie Rd.
Deland FL 32724

My brother-in-law gave me a bottle of Mountain Magic herbal tea to try as a preventive measure. I enjoyed the taste. Soon realized a 20 year stomach problem was gone,. and it gives me an all around better feeling. I am 60 years old and I work 7 days a week.

My nephew in Wisconsin learned he had cancer. He is unable to take Chemo because of other health problems. He takes your tea faithfully; one year later all is in remission. Our family also uses your organic sea salt; my wife used to have water retainage. No longer has a problem there. We enjoy your products and keep up the good work!

Robert W. Heath
9539 Stevenson Rd.
Fenwick MI 48834

I had prostate cancer. On August 10, 1994 I was given chemotherapy. I never told the doctor that I was taking Essiac and as a result the PSA rating went below 0 (zero). I took the combination for 15 months and when it held below zero I quit the chemotherapy. I am continuing taking the Essiac.

Paul Roche
East Haven, Connecticut

I have multiple sclerosis. My friend Kelly started me on Essiac. After three months I was able to put my crutches away. After a year, I walk with only a slight limp.

Barbara Johnson
Apopka, FL

I am in my fifties. It seems as if all my life I have had the flu at least once each year, and a bad cold for several times each year. It was like you could just automatically block out 1 to 2 months of each year when I would be laid up with the flu or a bad cold. I started taking Mountain Magic Essiac five years ago. Since that time I have not had the flu, and only had a cold once (I think that the cold was part of a detoxification process). I am sure that Essiac did this for me.

Mitchell Allen.
Orlando, Florida

My brother was diagnosed one year ago with very, very severe leukemia. His doctors gave him chemotherapy for four weeks. The chemo made him look deathly ill. My sister and I were appalled. He looked like death itself. This large man, who was over 6 feet tall, lay in his hospital bed in a fetal position, shaking from the chemotherapy.

The doctors told him that he would die in the hospital if he stayed, or he could go home and die. My sister is a nurse, and she was determined to save my brother. She knew of the herbal remedy for cancer called Essiac. She asked the doctor to approve bringing Essiac into the hospital to give to our brother. The doctor felt that there was nothing else he could do, so he paved the way with the medical authorities.

My brother began taking Essiac and 10 drops of Paul 'D Arco herbal formula each day, once in the morning, and once in the evening. His blood count was at 4,800 (10,000 is normal). Within one week of the Essiac treatment he was not only alive, his blood count was at 10,800. In one more week, his blood count was up to 14,000--4,000 higher than normal.

My brother began his Essiac treatments in August, 1992. He was so healthy by the next January that he and his wife went on a four month cruise around the world. It is now August 1993, and he is very healthy, active and robust. I have to withhold my name because I do not want a lot of people calling me about his experience. I love my brother very much, we are very close, and I just thank God for simple things like Essiac, and the people all over who prayed for his recovery.

Name Withheld By Request

I have a friend from West Virginia who has had rheumatoid arthritis for over 9 years. In May I gave her some of my Essiac. She liked it and began taking it regularily. Within 2 weeks she felt great relief from her pain. Within 2 months she could raise her arms full length over her head, something she had not been able to do for 9 years. She just went to Ireland to visit her relatives, and she took some Essiac with her to give to them.

Alice Bailey
Winter Springs, Florida

Several years ago, I escorted my mother to the outpatient clinic of a local hospital to have a small lump removed from her parotid gland on the left side of her face. What a shock when the doctors found advanced lymphoma cancer throughout her body. I began researching volumes of books looking for some unknown answer. A program of nutritional supplementation and natural food diet was begun, in addition to chiropractic care, positive thought, and humor therapy.

It was extremely tense as the doctors began chemotherapy. In fact, mother was taken to the emergency room six times the first month. Being 80, it was probably her strong heart that kept her alive and with me to tell her story today. Dancing and teaching others to stay well through dance has kept her going strong all her life.

Letters with prayers for her improved health poured in and a friend sent an article about "Essiac" tea. Hopeful that this herbal formula could somehow help, I went searching for the ingredients, brewed the tea, and added it to her growing list of nutritional supplements.

On Christmas Eve, 1992, three months after my mother's diagnosis of lymphoma, the doctors pronounced that my mother was not just in remission but cancer-free! While we will probably never know what cured her of this dreaded disease, we feel in our hearts that Essiac and nutrition played a major role.

J. Candy Arnold
Bellevue, Washington

Our family was devastated when my mother-in-law, Myrna, informed us that she had been diagnosed with cancer. In her case, it was ovarian cancer that had spread to the lymph glands and then into the lungs. It was diagnosed as inoperative, and the doctors told her to get her affairs in order. After a hysterectomy, they said, she would have about six months to live. The tumors in her lungs were too numerous to remove. My sister-in-law asked if there was some nutritional approach that might slow the progress of the disease. The doctor assured her there was none. But I nevertheless began to search for alternative remedies. By chance, my father heard a radio program where Essiac was explained.

The remedy was so simple and straightforward that I knew my mother-in-law could take it. She took a little each night. We held our breaths. The doctor and our nurse cousin told us not to get our hopes up. Yet, the weekly x-rays began indicating something they did not expect. Little by little the tumors in her lungs stabilized...and they began to diminish. The nursing staff at the doctor's office reacted in awe as week after week the tumors began disappearing, and her blood count returned to normal.

A little more than a year after beginning Essiac, the doctor called to tell Myrna that she was an official miracle. Her charts showed no indication of cancer in any system. To date, five years later, there has been no recurrence of cancer.

J.R. Kirkland
Washington

Where to Buy Your Essiac:

My longtime supplier is Natural Heritage Enterprises. Their website is www.remedies.net. Their product and service is the best. The ladies who man the telephone are loving and dedicated to helping their customers. Their prices are fair and their quality is excellent.

But the main reason that I recommend them is because of the extra qualities in their tea. They use "Structured water" to make their tea. This makes their tea by far the best, as you get the healing qualities of "structured water" along with the healing qualities of the tea. Just google "structured water" a discovery of Viktor Shauberger and Dr. Masaru Emoto, to find out about this valuable and amazing healing water.

Also, these people are healers first, and business people second. They are really dedicated to helping you. I like that.

They also give away free seven ebooks on healing that have proven helpful to me. Diabetes, arthritis, weight loss, women's beauty, ormus, sacred geometry for healing, anti-aging and longevity are among the topics. Very interesting stuff!

www.remedies.net

Printed in Great Britain
by Amazon